Mediterranean Diet

The 28-Day Kickstart Beginners Plan for a Rapid Weight Loss

Charles Kelso

Contents

Introduction

The Mediterranean diet is a time-tested and proven way to improve your overall health. Not only does this diet overload your taste buds with some of the tastiest foods in the world, it's also one of the most sustainable ways to lose weight, decrease inflammation, and live a healthier life.

The Mediterranean diet is one of the healthiest diets in existence. I wouldn't really call it a diet as much as it's a way of life. People living along the Mediterranean coast have been living this lifestyle for centuries. As a result, it has earned the reputation of being a powerful disease prevention tool.

So now let's look at some of the amazing benefits that come with this amazing new way of life.

1. Avoids Processed Foods and Sugar

Since the Mediterranean diet consists of natural foods like olive oil, legumes, fruits, and small portions of animal products, when contrasted to the Western diet, it's extremely low in sugar and free of artificial ingredients. When they want to eat something sweet, they eat fruit rather than processed snack cakes. Or they would use natural honey to sweeten their cup of tea.

Aside from vegetables and fruits, the Mediterranean diet also consists of a lot of fish. In fact, fish are a major staple of this lifestyle. While meat consumption is lower than most Western diets, you are not required to become a vegetarian. The idea is to remove those processed foods from your diet and replace them with healthier, natural alternatives.

2. You Will Lose Weight in a Healthy Way

If you are looking for an amazing way to lose weight in a healthy and sustainable way, then you have picked up the right book. As I said before, the Mediterranean diet is a lifestyle, so it can become a normal part of your life. There's no need to starve yourself to the brink of insanity. Its very nature leads to a natural reduction in fat intake, therefore leading to natural weight loss.

You can also mix and match this dieting plan with other changes. For example, if you want to mix in a low-carb lifestyle, then it's possible. If you want moderately higher protein because you want to build muscle mass, then you can do that as well. It's quite adaptive.

3. It Significantly Improves the Health of Your Heart

Numerous studies have shown that the Mediterranean diet is directly linked to a decrease in the risk of heart disease. That's because these foods are loaded with omega-3 fatty acids and monounsaturated fats.

Olive oil is a major ingredient in most recipes pertaining to the Mediterranean diet, and it has many tremendous benefits. One is that it helps to clear arteries and combat disease effects of oxidation and improves the endothelial function. But one thing that most people get wrong is that they believe that the lower their cholesterol, the better, but that's not really the case. You can actually have cholesterol levels that are too low. Fortunately, the Mediterranean diet promotes a healthy level of cholesterol. People who follow through with it do not struggle with cholesterol.

4. It's Known to Help Fight Cancer

The ratio of foods containing omega-3 and omega-6 fatty acids, in combination with the high amount of fiber you will consume on the Mediterranean diet has been shown in numerous studies as a biological mechanism to prevent cancer. Plant-based foods are central to this lifestyle, which protect from DNA damage and prevent cell mutation.

The fact is that cancer is still somewhat of a mystery, but what we do know is that living a healthy lifestyle will help prevent it. The Mediterranean diet reduces inflammation and will reduce oxidative stress.

5. It Helps Prevent and Can Even Treat Diabetes

Evidence shows us that the Mediterranean diet provides a host of anti-inflammatory benefits that will help you fight diseases related to inflammation, including type 2 diabetes. This lifestyle controls excess insulin, which in turn lowers our blood sugar levels.

Regulating our blood sugar levels is vastly important to living a healthier lifestyle. We're balancing a lot of whole foods into this plan so we find quality sources of protein and consume carbs that are low in sugar. That makes the body burn fat much more efficiently, and you will have more energy as a result. In short, a natural diet with fresh produce is a natural combater of diabetes.

6. Protects Your Cognitive Health
Choosing this lifestyle will actually help you preserve your memory, leading to an overall increase in your cognitive health. When the brain is not getting enough dopamine, we start to experience cognitive disorders like memory loss and a decrease in over thought processing.

Healthy fats are actually known to fight these cognitive disorders. Add in fresh veggies and you will counter all of the harmful toxins that are plaguing our diets right now. This also improves your mood.

7. Helps Relieve Stress
Finally, another of the main benefits of the Mediterranean diet is that it encourages you to eat foods that help reduce

inflammation. Everyone knows that stress can ruin your life. It can lead to all kinds of health problems, like obesity and high blood pressure.

The Mediterranean diet provides you with foods that promote a better mood, so you'll naturally reduce your stress. Additionally, this lifestyle also allows for red wine, which is healthy in moderation. The bottom line is that the Mediterranean diet will reduce your overall stress.

Follow These Tips for Success

Whatever your goals might be, it's important to create habits that help you along on your journey. In most cases, these habits are the difference between achieving your goals and failing. For the Mediterranean diet, these are some habits that you will need to develop in order to find success. If you can develop these into everyday habits, then you are tripling your chances of success!

Learn to Depend on More Than Willpower

Many people blame their dieting failures on a lack of willpower because it's the easiest excuse in the book. Willpower is never going to overpower your body's survival instincts, which is where cravings are created. That means it's important that you learn to depend on more than willpower. You need to take active steps to ensure that you are not tempted into submission.

In fact, people who base their dietary plans around willpower, rather than building a solid foundation for success, are far more likely to fail. Resisting temptations is much harder when it's right in front of you. So rather than relying on your willpower to keep you from grabbing that bag of chips from the pantry, make sure those chips are not there to begin with. If you find the vending machine at work too much of a temptation, then make sure you don't take cash to work. That way you can't use the machine.

Also, try removing stress from your life since it adds to temptation. Studies show that it's harder to resist unhealthy foods when you are stressed. Set a goal to be more consciously aware of your choices so that you can remove temptation whenever possible. That puts far less strain on your willpower.

Build a Foundation for Success
This habit builds on the last one because building a foundation for success on any diet requires you to remove any foods that do not support your new lifestyle. For example, if you toss out your sodas then you will not be tempted by them during those tough sugar cravings. If you prefer bottled water, then keep it on hand. Build a foundation that supports your success.

Another way to build this foundation is to set up a system so that you are more active throughout the day. Clean up an area of your home so that you can exercise. You can also take small steps like parking further away from the supermarket so that you have to walk a bit further. There are a lot of really simple things that you can do to become more active.

Realistic Goals Are Essential

A huge problem when making lifestyle changes comes from setting unrealistic goals. For instance, if you have been inactive for a lengthy period of time, then setting a goal to work out every day would be unrealistic. A more realistic goal would be to work out three days every week, and then work your way up from there. Always make sure your goal is achievable, then build up to bigger goals.

If a goal seems too difficult, one way to create confidence is to cut it in half. Then set dates to increase those goals. For instance, you might want to work out three days a week for the first month, and then increase it to four days per week.

Learn Portion Control

When following the Mediterranean diet, it's important that you learn to measure and control your portions. Most people look at a "portion" as the amount on their plate, but that's not the case. It all boils down to the number of calories you are consuming.

Furthermore, some foods are much denser in calories than others. Vegetables often contain fewer calories per serving than meat. You should learn to limit meals to one serving per food group. It can be difficult at first since we're all used to overeating, but once you develop this habit, your body will thank you!

Start Picturing Your Future Self
Have you stopped to consider where this journey is going to take you? What are your long-term goals? Are you trying to lose weight or just live a healthier lifestyle? Whatever the case, you should try to picture yourself the way you hope to be a year from now.

How do you look? How do you feel? Imagine your lifestyle the way you want it to be. Then use that image to create some positive affirmations about this new lifestyle. This will help you create a mindset that propels you towards being successful.

You Must Be Willing to Put in the Work
Humans are conditions to repeat the same actions until we take an active stance for change. In other words, if we just rely on our own inhibitions, then we're going to keep repeating the same mistakes. So if you are used to eating fast food every day, then that's what you are going to do until you take an active stance for change. Change takes work. Nothing in this book will help you if you are not willing to put in the work.

Introduction

New habits are going to take a lot of effort on your part. Post reminders, and write down lists to help you remember to make different choices.

Chapter 1
How Does the Mediterranean Diet Work?

Over the last half-century or so, the way we look at Mediterranean foods has changes. Most people imagine huge feasts with courses of pizza, lasagna, and endless bottles of wine. But the truth is that we have painted an inaccurate picture of the true Mediterranean lifestyle.

This diet is based on traditional fruits, olive oil, beans, and seafood. That's how the citizens living in southern Italy used to eat back when they boasted the lowest chronic disease rates in the world. The whole goal of the Mediterranean diet is to eat fresh foods while avoiding all of that processed junk that we find loitering around supermarkets.

These fresh foods will benefit you in a lot of different ways, as seen in the previous section. Plus they are quite delicious. The problem comes from changing diets, which is always a difficult change to make. I'm not going to sugar coat it and say that it's going to be easy because it's not. We have all become addicted to processed foods because they are so convenient.

Don't panic, though, because you do not have to make every change all at once. You can gradually work your way up to a healthier lifestyle. Plus, I promise that once you get used to eating fresh, whole foods, you will absolutely love this new lifestyle.

Some Myths Surrounding the Mediterranean Diet
There are a great number of misconceptions surrounding the Mediterranean diet and how it can lead to a healthier lifestyle. So let's look at some of those before moving on.

Myth #1: Following This Diet is Expensive
You will be creating meals out of lentils and/or beans and adding in whole grains and fresh vegetables. If you add everything up, the Mediterranean diet is actually cheaper than processed food.

Myth #2: The More Wine I Consume, The Healthier it Is
Wine, like so many other things in life, is healthy in moderation, but unhealthy if overindulged in. One glass of wine per day has a lot of amazing health benefits, but when you drink too much, you will start to experience negative effects that get worse as you drink more. In fact, anything more than two glasses of wine per day is bad for your heart.

Myth #3: Eating Large Bowls of Bread or Pasta is Okay
Western culture has a way of overexaggerating the Mediterranean diet with large servings of bread and pasta, but that's not what you should be doing. Pasta is normally just a side dish where you should only have up to a cup per meal.

The rest of the meal is based on salads, vegetables, and meats like fish. Maybe you can add in a slice of bread.

Myth #4: It's Only About the Food
Naturally, food choice is a huge part of living a healthier life, but there are other factors to the Mediterranean diet that simply cannot be overlooked. When Mediterranean's have a meal, they enjoy it with their family. It's a very special time for them. Enjoying a leisurely meal with others can greatly benefit your mental health and help you live a happier life. Furthermore, they also have a more physical and active lifestyle.

How to Change to the Mediterranean Diet

If you find the change in lifestyle intimidating, then know that you're not alone. Making changes to your life is not easy. Changing your eating habits over to the Mediterranean diet is challenging, so here are some tips to get you started. After this, we will start getting into more detail.

Eat a lot more veggies. Start off simple. Maybe a plate full of sliced tomatoes topped with feta cheese and drizzled with olive oil? Start loading your pizza with veggies rather than more meat. Salads are another great way to add vegetables into your diet. The key is to get into the habit of replacing meats with vegetables.

How Does the Mediterranean Diet Work?

<u>Stop skipping breakfast.</u> Fruits and whole grain foods are one of the best ways to start off your day. They give you a boost of energy while keeping you full into the afternoon.

<u>Eat more seafood.</u> Replace red meat with fish or shellfish. This one change will provide your brain and heart with a significant health boost.

<u>Go vegetarian at least one day per week.</u> Choose a day in the week to go completely meatless. Replace those meats with beans, whole grains, and vegetables. Once you get into the habit of a meat-free day, then you can try for two nights per week. That should be your end goal.

<u>Dairy should only be consumed in moderation.</u> You can still enjoy the occasional dairy product, but you will need to make sure you keep your saturated fat intake to less than ten percent of your daily calorie total.

<u>Choose the right desserts.</u> Rather than eating baked goods or other processed desserts, opt for fruit.

<u>Use only good fats.</u> Olive oil, sunflower seeds, and avocados are all amazing sources of fat. Stay away from vegetable oils and other processed fats when cooking.

Chapter 2
Foods to Eat on the Mediterranean Diet

First of all, there is no one way fits all approach to the Mediterranean diet. It's one of the most adaptive diets on the planet. So keep in mind that while this chapter will show you all of the basic foods that you'll consume on this diet, it is not set in stone. I just want to provide you with a few guidelines to help you start your journey.

Some of the Basics
Here is a quick glance at some of the basic foods that you should eat, as well as those you should avoid.

Eat These: Fruits, vegetables, seeds, legumes, potatoes, whole grains, fish, olive oil.

Eat Only in Moderation: Poultry, eggs, cheese, and yogurt.

Eat Rarely: Red meat.

Avoid These Foods at All Costs
Here is a quick glance at the foods that you should avoid at all costs.

Processed Sugar: This includes soda, candy, snack cakes, and any other form of processed sugar products. I cannot overemphasize how unhealthy these foods are for you.

Refined Grains: Any bread or pasta that is not made from whole grains should be avoided.

Trans Fats: These fats are found in processed foods and margarine. Make sure you do not use these.

Refined Oils: There are a ton of processed oils on the market. It's best to stick with extra-virgin olive oil so that you can avoid the unhealthy ones.

Processed Meat: Sausages and other processed meats are unhealthy due to all of the additives used.

Super High Processed Foods: These are usually hidden behind labels like "low fat" and "diet." If it looks like it was made in a factory, then it's probably going to be unhealthy.

Mediterranean Diet Approved Foods

Your new lifestyle should be based around these healthy choices. Just remember that this list is not set in stone. Basically, you should be okay if you stay away from processed foods.

Fresh Veggies: Vegetables are the staple of the Mediterranean diet. You are free to eat any vegetables you want, as long as they are fresh. Just keep in mind that green, leafy veggies are the best. It's also worth noting that you can choose frozen as long as you read the label to make sure there are no additives.

Seafood: Fish is another staple of the Mediterranean diet. Other shellfish like oysters, clams, trout, shrimp, and crab are also allowed.

Fresh Fruits: Fruits are another of the most important foods on the Mediterranean diet. Fresh fruits are always preferable, but you can use frozen, again, only if you carefully check the label to verify there are no additives.

Nuts and Seeds: Almonds, walnuts, hazelnuts, sunflower seeds, and almost all that fall under this category are a healthy choice.

Legumes: Peanuts, beans, and lentils are all amazing choices when following the Mediterranean diet.

Tubers: Sweet potatoes, potatoes, and other root-based vegetables are all fair game.

How Does the Mediterranean Diet Work?

Whole Grains: Any type of whole grain bread, pasta, brown rice, buckwheat, and whole oats are all a great addition to the Mediterranean diet.

Poultry: You should keep your poultry consumption in moderation. Turkey, chicken, and duck are allowed in limited quantities.

Dairy: Eggs, cheese, yogurt, and all other dairy products must be consumed in moderation.

Herbs and Spices: Herbs like garlic, rosemary, cinnamon, sage, and most other herbs and spices are okay. Just be sure to check the label to make sure there are no additives.

Healthy Fats: These include olive oil, olives, and avocados.

Some Important Notes About Food

The exact foods that you should include on the Mediterranean diet are a bit controversial since there are so many countries with such a variety of foods. The main takeaway is that there is no definitive list. With that in mind, your diet should be high in natural plant-based foods and low in animal foods. It's also recommended that you go meatless at least one day per week and that you eat seafood at least two times per week.

Some other things that factor into the Mediterranean lifestyle are physical activity, sharing meals as a family, and an overall enjoyment of life. It's not all about the food. Mindset is important with this new lifestyle.

What You Can Drink on the Mediterranean Diet
As with all diets in existence, water will be your go-to beverage. However, one glass of red wine every evening is an optional, yet beneficial, addition to this lifestyle, but you should not consume wine if you have a problem with alcoholism or anything like that.

You are also allowed to drink coffee and tea, as long as you do not add sugar to them.

Avoid all sugar-based drinks, including fruit juices, which are very high in sugar.

Amazing Snack Choices
Three meals per day is enough for those who choose to live the Mediterranean lifestyle. However, there will be times when you get hungry between meals. Staying hungry is never recommended since it will lead to powerful cravings, so here are some snacks that you can use to fill in those gaps.

> ➤ A handful of nuts should serve as an adequate snack.

➢ Whole fruit is another great choice.

➢ Carrots are a snack favorite of many people following this lifestyle.

➢ Berries can give you a small boost of energy to get you through the day.

➢ A small portion of leftovers from the night before can serve as a good snack. Just be sure not to overindulge.

➢ Greek yogurt makes for a delicious snack but should be eaten in moderation.

Sticking to the Mediterranean Diet While Eating Out

Unlike many other diets, it's actually easy to follow the Mediterranean diet when eating out. Most restaurants will have options that fall under this plan. Here are a few examples:

➢ Look through the menu to find a fish or seafood product to order as your main course.

➢ Some restaurants allow you the option to fry your foods in olive oil, but you have to request it.

➢ Ask if the bread and pasta is whole grain. If not, then you can just skip it.

The key is to know what foods to avoid, and do not order those.

Learn to Read Labels

Learning to understand food labels is one of the most important aspects of eating healthier. Companies are very good at hiding unhealthy foods behind fancy labels. Here is a step-by-step guide to help get you started.

Step 1: Serving Information

Always start with the serving information. Some companies will try to hide unhealthy foods behind small serving sizes. For example, 40 calories looks amazing until you realize that the serving size is only 1 tablespoon. Be sure that you pay close attention to the serving size to be sure that nothing is being hidden behind it.

Step 2: Calories Per Serving

After seeing the serving size, check out the total calories per serving. Then do the math, and add up the total calories per container to see the calorie total if you were to consume the whole package. Counting calories is important to living a healthier lifestyle. If you want to lose weight, you must put yourself at a calorie deficit.

How Does the Mediterranean Diet Work?

Step 3: Limit Certain Nutrients
You must limit the amount of saturated fat and sodium that you consume. You should also avoid trans-fat altogether. Always choose foods that limit these nutrients.

Step 4: Make Sure You Consume These Nutrients
Dietary fiber, protein, calcium, and other vitamins are all a necessary part of a healthy lifestyle. Make sure you are getting enough of these healthy nutrients by reading the food label.

Step 5: Learn About Daily Values
Finally, the daily values will show you the percentage of each nutrient based on a 2,000 calorie diet. As a general rule of thumb, if you want to eat less of a nutrient, then you will need to choose foods that have a daily value of five percent or less. If you want to get more of a nutrient, then aim for foods that have a daily value of at least 20 percent.

A Couple More Important Facts
Again, the daily values are based on a 2,000 calorie diet so you might need to lower those values depending on your dietary requirements. For instance, if you are looking to lose weight, then you will probably need to eat fewer than 2,000 calories.

If a food label says that a food contains 0g of trans-fat but has "partially hydrogenated oil" on the ingredient list, then it probably contains less than 0.5g. A nutrient that contains less than 0.5g can be labeled as 0g, but if you consume more than

1 serving, then it will quickly add up. Make sure you pay attention to the ingredient list.

The Mediterranean Diet Food Pyramid

The Mediterranean lifestyle follows a very specific food pyramid that is probably a little different than the one you're used to. Certain food groups are given priority while others should be consumed in moderation. Studies have shown that these foods are protective against the effects of certain chronic diseases.

In short, plant-based foods make up the largest chunk of this food pyramid so they should be consumed in greater proportions than the rest. You'll notice that all recipes found in this book are mostly comprised of plant-based foods. Here are some of the main takeaways from the Mediterranean food pyramid.

These Should Be Eaten Every Day

Your meals should be built around these three elements.

Whole Grains: You should consume at least one full serving of whole grains with every meal. These can be in the form of bread, pasta, rice, and couscous.

Vegetables: You should consume at least two servings of vegetables per meal. Including a variety of different vegetables ensures that you are getting all of the proper antioxidants and protective nutrients.

Fruits: You should consume at least two servings of fruit per day. You'll find that breakfast and late night desserts are your best options for eating fruit.

Make Sure You Drink Enough Water
I know it's not exactly a food group, but it's essential that you drink the right amount of water per day. Divide your weight in half to determine how many ounces of water you need to drink per day. Of course, this amount will change slightly depending on your age and the amount of physical activity you take part in every day.

Good hydration is important because it helps maintain balance within the body.

Consume These Foods in Moderation Daily
Here are some more important foods to the Mediterranean diet, but they should be eaten in moderation.

Dairy Products: You should consume at least one serving per day. Dairy products possess a lot of essential nutrients that contribute to good bone health and can also be an amazing source of healthy fats.

Olive Oil: There is a reason why olive oil can be found at the center of the Mediterranean food pyramid. This entire way of life revolves around it. Olive oil is highly nutritious, and its unique composition provides a much high resistance to cooking than other oils. It can also be used to make amazing homemade salad dressings. Just make sure you limit it to one tablespoon per meal.

Chapter 3
Shopping and Preparation

This chapter is going to focus on preparing your kitchen for this new lifestyle. There are a couple of small tips for shopping that I'm going to open with.

> ➢ Shop the perimeter of the supermarket because that's where all of the whole foods are located.

> ➢ Always make your decisions based on how processed the food is. The less processed, the better. Organic is the absolute best but also the most expensive.

One of the common things that I hear from individuals being part of a new dieting plan is that they "never eat junk food." While I would love to believe everyone, I know that realistically, what people say and what they do are sometimes different. Sure, some of them might be telling the truth, but I'm willing to bet that unless that took preventative steps to eliminate junk food from their homes, then they are falling prey to their cravings sometimes.

So the first step is to clear out the pantries and cupboards in order to remove temptation.

Clearing Out Your Kitchen

Start by getting rid of all of those really bad foods from your pantry. Throw away all of those sugary cereals and processed oatmeal packets. You should replace them with high fiber cereals like whole grain oatmeal and granola.

Throw away all of those prepackaged meals like Sloppy Joe mixes and Hamburger Helper. These are loaded with all kinds of unhealthy ingredients. There are much better choices.

Throw away all of those processed pastas and replace them with whole grain options. You will be able to make your own meals using higher quality ingredients. In many cases, it's actually cheaper than those prepackaged meals.

Make sure your pantry is stocked with everything you need to make fresh recipes. Some of these items include beans, whole-grain rice, whole wheat pasta, and even low-sodium chicken broth.

You should throw away all of those processed snacks like crackers, potato chips, and Little Debbie snack cakes. Replace them with nuts and fresh fruits. These should be your go to snacks foods.

Once you have cleaned out your cupboards, move on to the fridge. Let's start with the freezer. Almost all frozen dinners are unhealthy, so you should throw them away. If you need convenient meals, then it's possible to cook your own food, freeze it, and then heat it up in the microwave later. Soups are the best for this method. Then go through the fridge and throw away all of those processed foods, like "low fat" or "fat free" dressings. Highly processed foods like that are completely unhealthy. Sodas should also be tossed in the garbage. Fruit juices are just as bad.

Restock Your Kitchen with Healthy Foods
Once you have cleared out your kitchen of all of those unhealthy, junk foods, then you will need to restock it with healthier options. We're going to focus on whole grains, fruits, and other natural ingredients so that you can make the absolute best meals.

Fresh Vegetables: Broccoli, spinach, kale, carrots, onions, etc.
(Note: Try to put an emphasis on green, leafy vegetables)

Frozen Vegetables: You must read the label carefully to make sure no unhealthy additives are present.

Seafood: Shrimp, shellfish, salmon, tuna, trout, etc.

Fruits: Bananas, apples, oranges, grapes, pineapple, etc.

Berries: Strawberries, blueberries, blackberries, etc.

Whole Grains: Breads and pastas should always be whole grain.

Legumes: Beans and lentils will make up most of this category.

Nuts: Walnuts, almonds, cashews, etc.

Seeds: Sunflower seeds, pumpkin seeds, etc.

Condiments: Try sticking to sea salt since it's much healthier. Then there is pepper, turmeric, etc.

Other Healthy Foods: Potatoes, sweet potatoes, cheese, Greek yogurt, chicken (limited quantities), Omega-3 rich eggs, olives, extra virgin olive oil.

Once you have restocked your kitchen with healthier options, you will find that craving will no longer be able to tempt you into cheating because you have removed the unhealthy foods.

Chapter 4
Amazing Snack Choices

Snacks might be one of the most important aspects of following through with any dieting plan. Most people see the word "snacking" in a negative light, but I am here to tell you that it's actually quite important. This chapter will focus on showing you how to find healthy, Mediterranean-friendly snacks to add into your new lifestyle.

There are a number of reasons why snacking is an essential part of a diet. First of all, eating smaller meals boosts your metabolism, so you'll want to lower your portions with main meals. Therefore, you will need some pick-me-ups throughout the day. Snacking is how you keep your metabolism burning.

Just about everyone snacks throughout the day. The problem is that most people choose candy bars or chips as their snack of choice. What we're going to do is replace those with healthier, more delicious snacks.

Why Snacking is So Healthy
Again, snack foods have earned a bad reputation because of the bad habits that society has taught us. Most commercial snacks provide no nutritional value and throw our metabolism out of whack. That does not mean that the overall concept of

snacking is flawed. It just means that we have to find healthier alternatives.

Furthermore, when you go into a meal feeling intense hunger, then you are probably going to overeat--or worse–grab the first unhealthy food that catches your attention. Having a snack between meals prevents this from becoming an issue. With the Mediterranean diet, choosing a snack that's whole grain is a perfect choice since complex carbohydrates are digested slowly.

Snacks are also a great way to add more specific nutrients into your diet. For instance, you can boost your potassium intake by eating a banana as a snack. Or you can increase your calcium intake by consuming a dairy product.

Ideal snacks should be approximately 200 calories or less.

Some Amazing Mediterranean Diet Snack Choices
Since the Mediterranean diet focuses on fresh, whole grain foods, then it's obvious that snacks should also be based around these types of foods. Here are five amazing choices, but feel free to experiment to find your own.

Hummus Dip with Raw Vegetables
Calories: 130

This is a chickpea-based dip that makes for an amazing snack. It's made using olive oil, is high in fiber, and has enough unsaturated fat and protein to satisfy your hunger for much longer than the traditional unhealthy snack. You can then dip your veggies into this dip to add in some important nutrients.

Unsalted Nuts (25g.)
Calories: 152 (changes based on the nut)

While nuts do contain a certain amount of fat, it's not enough to throw you off of your healthy lifestyle. Nuts are an amazing snack that are very high in protein, so they will keep you full for a long period of time. Furthermore, they provide fiber and other important nutrients. Almonds tend to be the best choice since they contain the most nutrients. Just make sure that you stick to a small handful, since nuts are loaded with calories.

Mediterranean-Friendly Salad
Calories: 107

This snack consists of 1 tomato with 25g of low fat feta cheese and 1 tablespoon of olive oil. This salad is a quick and delicious snack that is loaded with essential nutrients. Tomatoes alone contain an important antioxidant that actually has the potential to reverse cell damage. Furthermore, they contain a lot of vitamin A and C. When you pair this amazing food with feta cheese, you get an added boost of protein. The olive oil also adds healthy fat, leading to a delicious and ling-lasting afternoon snack.

Fruit and Dip
Calories: 147

One cup of fresh fruit and a half-cup of low fat yogurt dip makes for an amazing snack. You will need to slice up some fruit into pieces and then dip them in the low-fat yogurt. This is one of the most delicious snacks you can find. Plus, it provides a lot of essential nutrients like vitamins, fiber, and calcium. This snack is also perfect for parties!

Tuna and Crackers
Calories: 205

Use four whole wheat crackers and a small can of tuna for an amazing snack that's extremely high in protein. Oily fish are a staple of the Mediterranean diet, so by combining this with whole grain crackers, you are creating a highly nutritious snack. You are going to get an amazing dose of Omega-3 fatty acids and enough protein to keep you from getting hungry.

Chapter 5
Tracking Your Food and Calorie Intake

Tracking your food and calorie intake is an important part of living a healthier lifestyle. Research has proven time and time again that those who do not track their food tend to fail at dieting. Those who do keep track are far more likely to successfully reach their goals.

Fortunately, counting calories is not that difficult of a task in today's high tech world. There are a ton of useful websites and apps that will help you log each meal easily, giving you an easy platform to keep track of your daily calories.

We are going to look at five of the best calorie counters. These are all accessible on their website and have apps that can be downloaded to any Android or iPhone.

#1: My Fitness Pal
MyFitnessPal might be the most popular food tracking software on the planet right now. It allows you to keep track of your weight and shows you a recommended daily calorie intake based on your goals. The program operates flawlessly and contains amazing food diaries and exercise logs.

If using the website, you can look at a clear picture of the calories that you've consumed throughout any given day. More importantly, it helps you stay within your limits. It even goes as far as to show you how many calories you have burned through exercise!

You can even use a fitness tracking device and link it to MyFitnessPal for an automated way of keeping track of your daily activity.

You will also get support in chat forums that can help keep you motivated. Here, users share recipes, tips, and even personal success stories.

MyFitnessPal boasts an impressive database of over five million different foods and even allows you to program custom recipes and foods. It can even save your favorite meals so you can log them quickly.

Another amazing tool is that MyFitnessPal actually has a barcode scanner built into the system, so you can scan a lot of packaged foods to get the nutritional information automatically!

You will be able to see each day as a pie chart, showing you a breakdown of carbs, protein, and fat consumed each day. You are also able to make notes, which is a great way to document how you are feeling throughout the day. That way, you can go back and see the correlation of your mood in reaction to the foods you were eating.

While MyFitnessPal does offer a free version, if you want to unlock all of the premium benefits, then you will have to pay $49.99 per year. It's an investment that is well worth the payoff though!

Advantages

➤ MyFitnessPal boasts the largest database of all food tracking programs, and it also includes a lot of restaurant foods.

➤ You can download recipes online and then calculate their calorie content.

➤ There is a "quick add" option that allows you to input details about certain meals without having to add details. This is perfect when you're limited on time.

Disadvantages

➤ You will have to double-check recipes since most of them are uploaded by other users. There could also be multiple entries of the same food.

> Serving sizes that are present in the database are sometimes difficult to edit, making it a bit harder to judge your own servings if they are smaller or larger.

#2: Lose It!

Lose It! is another amazing food tracking program that makes it easy to record your food and exercise. You are even able to connect several fitness devices to this program, much like with MyFitnessPal.

This amazing program will create a list of personalized recommendations based on your weight, height, age, and your personal fitness goals. It will then track all of your calories on the homepage.

Lose It! also has a comprehensive food database, though not as large as MyFitnessPal. But the food diary is much simpler to use, and it's very easy to add new foods. It also has a barcode scanner for packaged foods. If you tend to eat the same food repeatedly, then it will be saved so you can easily find it under a quick entry.

You are able to quickly look at a graph of your weight changes both daily and weekly. They also have an active community where you can find support. You can even take part in specific challenges or make up your own!

While this app is free to use, you can set more goals and record more information by paying a yearly premium membership fee of $39.99.

Advantages

> ➤ Lose It has a comprehensive database loaded to the brim with foods, grocery stores, and popular restaurants. Unlike MyFitnessPal, these are all verified by a team of experts.

> ➤ You can set personal reminders to help you remember to log your meals and snacks.

Disadvantages

> ➤ It's difficult to keep track of the nutritional value of homemade meals and recipes.

> ➤ Lose It! can be a bit difficult to navigate.

> ➤ You are not able to track macronutrients like vitamins and minerals.

#3: SparkPeople

We come to another full-featured food tracker that helps you keep up with nutrition, activities, and personal health goals. The food diary is pretty simple, and if you happen to eat a lot of the same foods, then you can simply copy/paste entries.

Below every daily entry, you can see the total calorie count. There is also the ability to view this information as a pie chart, which would break down calories, carbs, protein, and fat.

SparkPeople also makes it easy to add recipes. There is even a barcode scanner so that you can register packaged foods relatively easily.

There is a massive community right at your fingertips so you can find support. What makes this community so different though is that experts will post health related articles to help you on your journey.

While the free version of this app boasts one of the largest databases in the world, you will have to upgrade to premium in order to gain access to many of the other features.

Advantages

> The website provides more resources than any other program of its type.

Disadvantages

> Since there is so much information included on this website, new users are sometimes overwhelmed.

> ➤ Content is spread out over multiple apps based on different topics. It can be quite confusing.

#4: Cron-o-Meter

Cron-o-Meter helps you keep track of your food intake by providing exact serving sizes, nutritional information, and an amazing exercise database. There is even a feature that helps pregnant women plan their diet around their pregnancy.

You can also tell this program what diet you are following and it will make macronutrient recommendations for you. This is a cool feature, but not really necessary on the Mediterranean diet since we're worried more about calories.

Cron-o-Meter also provides a very simple food diary that is designed for beginners. Below that diary is a chart that gives you a breakdown of your total calories consumed. It also allows you to track macronutrients.

The app does cost $2.99, so that is one of the disadvantages.

<u>Advantages</u>

> ➤ This app is designed for beginners, so it's extremely easy to use.

> ➤ Cron-o-Meter allows you to sync data from other health programs. For example, you can import your weight,

body fat percentage, and sleep habits from other programs.

➢ It keeps track of all micronutrients.

Disadvantages

➢ It does not divide food entries into separate meals.

➢ The only way to add homemade foods is through the website. You cannot do it within the app itself. However, once you add it on the website, then it's available on the app.

➢ There is no social community of users for support.

#5: FatSecret

FatSecret is a neat little free calorie counter that includes an exercise log, built-in recipes, and a food diary. It also has a barcode scanner that you can use to scan packaged foods.

Your total calorie intake is shown on the homepage. You'll also be able to see the exact breakdown of carbs, protein, and fat. Not that this information is important on the Mediterranean diet, but it's still a useful tool. You'll mainly be concerned with calorie intake.

You can even look at a detailed monthly review to see how many calories were consumed on each day, a feature that's convenient for tracking your overall goals. What makes FatSecret so appealing is its user-friendly interface.

You'll also find a very friendly community where users will support each other by swapping recipes, providing guidance, and even sharing their stories.

Advantages

- ➢ This easy-to-use app has a comprehensive database of foods and grocery stores.

- ➢ All food information that is provided by other users is highlighted, so you know which entries to double-check.

Disadvantages

- ➢ It does not possess some of the more complex reports that other food tracking programs provide.

Keeping a Written Food Journal

If apps are not appealing to you, then you can always keep track of your food intake the old-fashioned way. The truth is that you must track your food if you want any hope of being successful. This is the one step that can either make or break your success.

A food journal shows you exactly what you are eating and provides a clear picture of your daily consumption. Therefore, you will be able to adjust your eating habits in a healthier way.

> ➢ Write down what you eat and drink immediately. This includes water, so you can be sure you're drinking enough of it.

> ➢ Write down your activity while eating. For example, are you working, watching television, or driving?

> ➢ Try to describe why you ate. Was it hunger, or were you eating because you were emotional?

> ➢ Always be honest with yourself. Remember, no one will see this journal but you.

Chapter 6
Exercise

Including exercise in any dieting plan will drastically improve it. One of the staples of the Mediterranean lifestyle is being active. But if you're like most people, the word exercise can be quite intimidating. However, I'm going to make this extremely easy for you. This chapter will list several exercises that are designed specifically for beginners.

These beginner-level exercises are perfect in combination with the Mediterranean diet. They promote weight loss and better health. In fact, if you have ever tried exercising only to find that it was too much, then you will love these workouts. Our goal here is to build confidence and show you that exercise does not have to be intimidating. Once you have developed better habits, then you might be able to take it up a notch.

Are you ready to get started?

Benefits of Exercising

Here's some motivation for you. Beginners who start an exercise routine are going to experience a lot of added benefits alongside of their dieting plan. We're going to focus on low-intensity sessions that will actually help you burn more calories. As long as you keep your calorie intake at a deficit, you will lose weight.

Our bodies were meant to be active, but the problem is that many of us do not have a naturally active lifestyle. So we need to take the initiative and add it into our lives. The truth is that exercise does not have to be extreme. It's more about getting your metabolism burning than anything. These easy workouts will help you:

- ➢ Build confidence
- ➢ Establish better habits
- ➢ Develop tighter muscles
- ➢ Sleep better
- ➢ Lower your stress levels
- ➢ Burn more calories
- ➢ Lose weight

With that said, these exercises will improve your health.

There are a lot of medical benefits to exercise as well, but most media focus on high-intensity workouts. But low-intensity sessions remain the cornerstone of many weight loss programs. This includes people suffering from type 2 diabetes and high blood pressure.

Beginner's Workouts That Can be Done at Home

You have a lot to gain from getting into the habit of performing these easy exercises. The key is to perform some form of physical activity at least once per day. You can start out by setting a short-term goal of three exercises per week, and then gradually work your way up until you are exercising at least once per day.

The exact exercise you choose is not as important as the fact that you need to be active. You just need to be consistent. But here are some simple exercises that will help get you started.

Dancing: This is super simple. Just put on some great music, and dance for at least 15 minutes. It's that simple.

Online Exercises: Just open up YouTube, and find some online workouts. Many of them are super easy and perfect for beginners. Plus, you get the added benefit of exercising in the comfort of your own home.

Bodyweight Training: There is no need to invest in any gym equipment to build stronger muscles. You can spend 15 minutes per day doing simple bodyweight training. Pushups, squats, and lunges are all great examples of easy exercises that you can try.

Simple Exercises Away from Home

Exercising away from home actually comes with some unique perks. There are certain stress-relieving benefits to breathing fresh air and enjoying time away from home. Here are a few beginners' exercises that you can try:

Swimming: Swimming is the absolute best cardio workout that you can perform. It doesn't put stress on your joints like jogging does, and it provides the same benefits. So find a local pool and dive in!

Biking: Here is another time-honored form of exercise that is quite enjoyable. Just get on a bike and cruise around the neighborhood for 15 to 20 minutes.

Walking: You can always opt to go for a walk, which has a ton of benefits includes the fact that it relieves stress. You should try to walk for 30 minutes at a time.

There really are a lot of choices for beginners here, so it's up to you. Just be sure that you're being active for at least 15 minutes every day. What's important here is that you develop the habit of being active every day.

Chapter 7
Stay Motivated with the Mediterranean Diet

Sometimes staying motivated when it comes to making healthier choices can be quite difficult. Why else do you think there are so many failed New Year's resolutions made every year? Fortunately, there are ways that you can make sure that you stay motivated to make this important change to your life.

First of all, the most powerful motivator is to have friends and family who support your goals. When your social network starts tempting you with bad choices, then that can be a problem. Fortunately, you can find online networks who can provide the support you need to stay motivated. When people share common goals, they tend to accomplish more together.

Give Yourself a Pep Talk

Pep talks might seem silly to some people, but I promise you that they are powerful and will infuse you with a lot of positive energy. You should channel this power every day and tell yourself something positive every day. Use that time to reaffirm why you are trying to be healthier. Again, it seems silly at first until you realize just how powerful this method can be. This is a lesson that's taught by all of the top life coaches.

Find a Few Virtual Friends

Technology makes it easier than ever to connect with people from around the world. It's actually not that difficult to find people who share common goals. SparkPeople is a great online community where you can find people with health and fitness goals. Get out there and start chatting with people. Make some virtual friends and motivate each other.

Find Ways to Surround Yourself with Success

There is a saying that goes "misery loves company." Well the exact same thing can be said about happiness and success. Why do you think that health forums are so popular? People who are trying to change their lives for the better are often forced to overcome a lot of obstacles along the way. That's why it's so beneficial to have support during the most difficult of times. Surrounding yourself with others who are motivated to be successful will help lift you through those difficult times. It will keep you motivated in ways that nothing else can.

Don't Be Afraid to Pat Yourself on the Back

Even if no one else knows about one of your major achievements, that doesn't mean that you should not acknowledge it. Celebrate your achievements. Did you meet your first weight loss goal? Then consider treating yourself to a new outfit. Did you meet a huge exercise goal? Then give yourself a few words of encouragement. Visual reminders will help you stay motivated on those days when you might not be as motivated as you'd like.

Challenge Yourself

Competition is healthy and has a powerful motivational effect on you. You can either create challenges for yourself or join a forum like SparkChallenge to get that extra push. You should make sure that challenges you accept are aligned with your goals. Plus you get support, which we have already established is a powerful motivator.

Check in Every Week

Just because your friends might not fully support your new health goals doesn't mean that you are doomed to failure. You will find online friends who will support you. With that said, you should make it a point to schedule weekly check-ins with these people to discuss your successes and failures. This will help you stay on track and provides support for those weeks when you might have messed up.

Get Involved

If you happen to be new to the area, then you might have trouble finding an in-person support group. That means you'll have to get out there and take the initiative. Join a gym or join local meetings to find people with similar goals. You can even use Facebook to find people in your community. Don't be afraid to reach out to them.

Your Pet Can be Motivational

For example, your dog will not turn down the opportunity to get out of the house for a walk. Therefore, if you have a dog and have been just taking him/her into the back yard to use the potty, then take a trip around the block instead. Or go outside and play fetch with your dog. Pets can be extraordinarily motivational.

Keep a Journal

Documenting your goals and struggles is one of the best ways to keep yourself moving forward. We all have struggles and setbacks. Stumbling is not a negative thing as long as we learn from it. While many people have turned to digital journals or blogging as their form of journaling, you can always take an old-fashioned approach and go pen to paper. What's important is that you document your entire journey so that you can stay motivated to continue.

Reward Yourself

Don't do all of that work for free. Make sure that you have a reward system in place so that you are getting something in return for meeting your goals. An example of a reward system is to budget a specific amount of money to splurge once you meet a specific goal.

You should take this further by rewarding yourself for meeting weekly goals too. Just make sure that you're not rewarding yourself with unhealthy foods–a mistake that a lot of people make. Your rewards should align with your overall goals.

Final Thoughts
Learn to Master the Mediterranean Diet

As you have seen throughout this book, the Mediterranean diet is based around the foods that people ate in countries that border the Mediterranean Sea back in the '60s. That is the basis for the name. The concept is based around the fact that these countries experienced exceptional health during this time. Their risk of heart disease was much lower, and they experienced much happier lives.

By this point, you already have a great plan to begin this amazing journey, so now it's just a matter of mastering it. Here are some tips to help you do just that.

Nuts Should Be Your Go-To Snack
You should replace those candy bars and bags of chips with small packages of nuts. One of the most important parts of the Mediterranean diet is to make your own meals. That includes preparing your own snacks. Replace the candy bar in your desk drawer with a can of nuts, and when it you need a snack, eat a small palm full of them. You can also enjoy fruit for a snack if you're in the mood for something sweeter.

Final Thoughts

Eat Fruit Every Day

Fruit is considered nature's candy. It's healthy and will satisfy those sugar cravings you have between meals. Also, berries are a great morning snack because they have energy boosting properties. Many people who follow the Mediterranean diet choose fruit as their go-to breakfast.

Plan Meals Ahead of Time

You should plan out your meals before you go grocery shopping so that you know exactly what to buy. Plus, it will keep you from buying a bunch of junk that will just clutter your kitchen. In fact, planning meals ahead of time is a staple to success on any dieting plan. Spend some time over the weekend to plan out meals for the following week, and base your shopping list around those meals. This includes planning for snacks. Meal planning itself can drastically change your life for the better!

Start Eating More Fish

This is one of the areas where so many people mess up when trying the Mediterranean diet. They don't eat enough fish. Seafood is one of the most important foods on the Mediterranean diet. Yes, it's more expensive when compared to the standard red meat and poultry products, but it possesses nutrients that hold a lot of amazing benefits. Try to plan at least three meals per week around fish like salmon, cod, or tilapia.

Use Olive Oil Instead of Butter

The Mediterranean diet promotes the use of olive oil as a replacement for all other types of oils, including butter. When possible, swap out the butter in certain recipes with olive oil. It's an amazing cooking ingredient and can even be used to make some of the best homemade salad dressings. That brings us to...

Start Making Your Own Salad Dressings

Olive oil is a great base for salad dressings. You should start making your own rather than buying sugar-loaded manufactured dressing. It's actually pretty easy to make your own dressing and much healthier.

Enjoy One Glass of Wine per Day

One glass of wine per day is recommended for those following the Mediterranean diet. Just remember that drinking too much will actually be bad for your health. But in limited quantities, wine has a ton of beneficial effects.

Four-Week Mediterranean Meal Plan

Meal Plan Introduction

Now we're going to take a closer look at an amazing four-week meal plan to help get you started. This will make it much easier to get you started on your new Mediterranean lifestyle. As you know, my goal with this book has been to make it as easy as possible for you to swap over to a healthier lifestyle.

1. I have mentioned this several times throughout this book and will mention it again. You must carefully read labels before you add any food to a recipe to make sure that it's healthy. Some manufacturers will hide unhealthy foods behind fancy labels, but they cannot hide the ingredients and nutritional values from those of us who know where to look.

2. Some meals in this plan will leave you with leftovers so you don't have to cook every day. This can be a lifesaver for those of you who are constantly busy.

3. You should always track your daily calories, and make sure you are under your recommended count if your goal is to lose weight. Just remember that you will only lose weight if you are at a calorie deficit.

4. Exercise is an essential part of the Mediterranean lifestyle. However, if you are physically active throughout the day then

Final Thoughts

you do not necessarily have to follow through with an exercise
plan.

Week 1

Monday

Breakfast: Breakfast Quinoa

Lunch: Medley Salad

Afternoon Snack: One piece of fruit

Dinner: Pan-Seared Scallops with Pepper and Onions, Fruit

Tuesday

Breakfast: One piece of fruit

Lunch: Mediterranean Wrap

Afternoon Snack: Palm full of nuts (your choice of nut)

Dinner: Pan-Seared Scallops with Pepper and Onions (Leftover from Monday), fruit

Wednesday

Breakfast: Almond, Banana Oatmeal

Lunch: Mediterranean Wrap (Leftover from Tuesday)

Afternoon Snack: One piece of fruit

Dinner: Mediterranean Chicken with Eggplant, fruit

Thursday

Breakfast: One piece of fruit

Final Thoughts

Lunch: Pasta Chickpea Salad

Afternoon Snack: Palm full of nuts (your choice of nut)

Dinner: Mediterranean Chicken with Eggplant (leftover from Wednesday), Fruit

Friday

Breakfast: Grilled Banana and Peanut Butter Sandwich

Lunch: Pasta Chickpea Salad (leftover from Thursday)

Afternoon Snack: One piece of fruit

Dinner: Orzo and Chicken Salad in Red Pepper Cups, fruit

Saturday

Breakfast: One piece of fruit

Lunch: Orzo and Chicken Salad in Red Pepper Cups (leftover from Friday)

Afternoon Snack: Palm full of Nuts (your choice of nut)

Dinner: Greek Potatoes, Fruit

Sunday

Breakfast: Egg White Omelet

Lunch: Spaghetti Squash

Afternoon Snack: Palm full of nuts (your choice of nut)

Dinner: Spaghetti Squash (leftover from lunch), fruit

Week 2

Monday

Breakfast: <u>Almond, Banana Oatmeal</u>

Lunch: <u>Black Bean Hummus</u>

Afternoon Snack: One piece of fruit

Dinner: <u>Brown Rice Salad</u>, fruit

Tuesday

Breakfast: One piece of fruit

Lunch: <u>Brown Rice Salad</u> (leftover from Monday)

Afternoon Snack: Palm full of nuts (your choice of nut)

Dinner: <u>Penne with Yogurt-Tahini Sauce</u>, fruit

Wednesday

Breakfast: <u>Breakfast Quinoa</u>

Lunch: <u>Penne with Yogurt-Tahini Sauce</u> (Leftover from Tuesday)

Afternoon Snack: One piece of fruit

Dinner: <u>Sicilian Lemon Chicken</u>, fruit

Thursday

Breakfast: One piece of fruit

Lunch: <u>Sicilian Lemon Chicken</u> (leftover from Wednesday)

Afternoon Snack: Palm full of nuts (your choice of nut)

Dinner: <u>Fish Soup</u>, fruit

Friday

Breakfast: <u>Egg White Omelet</u>

Lunch: <u>Tuna and Avocado Tapas</u>

Afternoon Snack: One piece of fruit

Dinner: <u>Fish Soup</u>, fruit

Saturday

Breakfast: One piece of fruit

Lunch: <u>Tuna and Avocado Tapas</u> (leftover from Friday)

Afternoon Snack: Palm full of nuts (your choice of nut)

Dinner: <u>Fish Soup</u> (leftover from Friday), fruit

Sunday

Breakfast: <u>Grilled Banana and Peanut Butter Sandwich</u>

Lunch: <u>Tilapia Feta Florentine</u>

Afternoon Snack: Palm full of nuts (your choice of nut)

Dinner: <u>Tilapia Feta Florentine</u> (leftover from lunch), fruit

Week 3

Monday

Breakfast: Egg White Omelet

Lunch: Mediterranean Wrap

Afternoon Snack: One piece of fruit

Dinner: Spinach and Feta Pita Bake, fruit

Tuesday

Breakfast: One piece of fruit

Lunch: Spinach and Feta Pita Bake (leftover from Monday)

Afternoon Snack: Palm full of nuts (your choice of nut)

Dinner: Pan-Seared Scallops with Pepper and Onions, fruit

Wednesday

Breakfast: Grilled Banana and Peanut Butter Sandwich

Lunch: Tahini Spinach

Afternoon Snack: One piece of fruit

Dinner: Pan-Seared Scallops with Pepper and Onions (leftover from Tuesday), fruit

Thursday

Breakfast: One piece of fruit

Lunch: <u>Tahini Spinach</u> (leftover from Wednesday)

Afternoon Snack: Palm full of nuts (your choice of nut)

Dinner: <u>Tuna and Avocado Tapas</u>, fruit

Friday

Breakfast: <u>Almond, Banana Oatmeal</u>

Lunch: <u>Tuna and Avocado Tapas</u> (leftover from Thursday)

Afternoon Snack: One piece of fruit

Dinner: <u>Whole Wheat Pizza</u>, fruit

Saturday

Breakfast: One piece of fruit

Lunch: <u>Sicilian Lemon Chicken</u>

Afternoon Snack: Palm full of nuts (your choice of nut)

Dinner: <u>Whole Wheat Pizza</u> (leftover from Friday), fruit

Sunday

Breakfast: <u>Breakfast Quinoa</u>

Lunch: <u>Sicilian Lemon Chicken</u> (leftover from Saturday)

Afternoon Snack: Palm full of nuts (your choice of nut)

Dinner: <u>Sicilian Lemon Chicken</u> (leftover from Saturday), fruit

Week 4

Monday

Breakfast: Almond, Banana Oatmeal

Lunch: Mediterranean Bean Salad

Afternoon Snack: One piece of fruit

Dinner: Parma Wrapped Chicken with Mediterranean Vegetables, fruit

Tuesday

Breakfast: One piece of fruit

Lunch: Medley Salad

Afternoon Snack: Palm full of nuts (your choice of nut)

Dinner: Parma Wrapped Chicken with Mediterranean Vegetables (leftover from Monday), fruit

Wednesday

Breakfast: Egg White Omelet

Lunch: Pasta Chickpea Salad

Afternoon Snack: One piece of fruit

Dinner: Spanish Cod, fruit

Thursday

Breakfast: One piece of fruit

Lunch: <u>Mediterranean Greek Salad</u>

Afternoon Snack: Palm full of nuts (your choice of nut)

Dinner: <u>Spanish Cod</u> (leftover from Wednesday), fruit

Friday

Breakfast: <u>Breakfast Quinoa</u>

Lunch: <u>Tuna and Avocado Tapas</u>

Afternoon Snack: One piece of fruit

Dinner: <u>Melitzanes Imam</u>, fruit

Saturday

Breakfast: One piece of fruit

Lunch: <u>Tuna and Avocado Tapas</u> (leftover from Friday)

Afternoon Snack: Palm full of nuts (your choice of nut)

Dinner: <u>Melitzanes Imam</u> (leftover from Friday), fruit

Sunday

Breakfast: <u>Grilled Banana and Peanut Butter Sandwich</u>

Lunch: <u>Vegetable and Bread Soup</u>

Afternoon Snack: Palm full of nuts (your choice of nut)

Dinner: <u>Vegetable and Bread Soup</u> (leftover from lunch), fruit

Recipes

Recipe List

Almond, Banana Oatmeal

Servings: 1

Ingredients

- ✓ 1 Small banana
- ✓ 1 Cup almond milk
- ✓ 1 Tbsp. honey
- ✓ 1 Tsp. almond extract
- ✓ ¼ Tsp. ground cinnamon
- ✓ Pinch of sea salt
- ✓ ½ Cup rolled oats

Directions

1. Mash half of the banana into a saucepan.

2. Whisk together almond milk, honey, almond extract, cinnamon, and salt along with the mashed banana until it's smooth. Bring this new mixture to a boil.

3. Stir in oats and reduce heat to medium-low. Simmer until the oats have become tender and are consistent with your preference. This takes approximately 5 minutes.

4. Move oatmeal to a bowl. Top with cinnamon if desired.

5. Top oatmeal with the remainder of banana.

Nutritional Information

Calories: 385

Fat: 6g.

Carbs: 77g.

Protein: 8g.

Black Bean Hummus

Servings: 3

Ingredients

- ✓ 1 Can of black beans (15 Oz.), drained. Save liquid.
- ✓ 1 Clove of garlic
- ✓ 2 Tbsp. lemon juice
- ✓ 1 ½ Tbsp. tahini
- ✓ ¾ Tsp. ground cumin
- ✓ ½ Tsp. salt
- ✓ ¼ Tsp. cayenne pepper
- ✓ ¼ Tsp. paprika
- ✓ 10 Greek olives

Directions

1. Mince garlic in a food processor.

2. Add black beans, 2 Tbsp. of the saved liquid, 2 tablespoons lemon juice, tahini, 1/2 teaspoon cumin, 1/2 teaspoon salt, and 1/8 teaspoon cayenne pepper. Process until smooth.

3. Add more seasoning and liquid to taste.

4. Garnish with paprika and Greek olives.

Nutritional Information

Calories: 81

Fat: 3g.

Carbs: 10g.

Protein: 4g.

Breakfast Quinoa

Servings: 1

Ingredients

- ✓ ¼ Cup raw almonds, raw
- ✓ 1 Tsp. ground cinnamon
- ✓ 1 Cup quinoa
- ✓ 2 Cups milk

- ✓ 1 Tsp. sea salt
- ✓ 1 Tsp. vanilla extract
- ✓ 2 Tbsp. honey
- ✓ 2 Dried pitted dates, chopped
- ✓ 5 Dried apricots, chopped

Directions

1. Toast almonds using a skillet on medium. This takes approximately 3-5 minutes. Place almonds to the side.

2. Combine cinnamon and quinoa in a sauce pan, and heat on medium until thoroughly warmed. Add milk and sea salt to the saucepan. Bring to a boil and reduce heat to low. Place lid on saucepan and simmer for 15 minutes.

3. Mix vanilla, honey, dates, apricots, and half the almonds with the quinoa mixture. Top with the rest of the almonds before serving.

Nutritional Information

Calories: 327

Fat: 8g.

Carbs: 54g.

Protein: 12g.

Brown Rice Salad

Servings: 2

Ingredients

- ✓ 1 ½ Cup brown rice
- ✓ 3 Cups water
- ✓ 1 Red bell pepper, sliced into thin pieces
- ✓ 1 Cup frozen green peas
- ✓ ½ Cup raisins
- ✓ ¼ chopped sweet onion
- ✓ ¼ Cup Kalamata olives, chopped
- ✓ ½ Cup vegetable oil
- ✓ ¼ Cup balsamic vinegar
- ✓ 1 ¼ Tsp. Dijon mustard
- ✓ Dash of sea salt
- ✓ Dash of pepper
- ✓ ¼ Cup feta cheese

Directions

1. Bring water and brown rice to a boil on high. Reduce heat and simmer until rice is fully cooked.

2. Mix red bell pepper, peas, raisins, onion, and olives in a bowl.

3. In another bowl, whisk vegetable oil, vinegar, and mustard to create the dressing.

4. Mix together vegetables, vinegar, rice, and dressing. Use sea salt and pepper to season.

5. Top with feta cheese.

Nutritional Information

Calories: 451

Fat: 24g.

Carbs: 55g.

Protein: 7g.

Easy Mediterranean Fish

Servings: 4

Ingredients

- ✓ 4 Halibut fillets, 6 Oz. each
- ✓ 1 Tbsp. Greek seasoning
- ✓ 1 Chopped large tomato
- ✓ 1 Chopped onion
- ✓ 1 Jar of pitted kalamata olives
- ✓ ¼ Cup capers
- ✓ ¼ Cup olive oil

✓ 1 Tbsp. lemon juice
✓ Dash of black pepper

Directions

1. Preheat oven to 350 degrees.

2. Place the fillets one a sheet of aluminum foil and use the Greek seasoning to season them.

3. Mix together tomato, onion, olives, capers, olive oil, lemon juice, salt, and pepper in a bowl.

4. Use a spoon to spread the tomato mix over the fillets. Seal all edges of the aluminum foil to create a packet. Place it onto a baking sheet.

5. Bake for approximately 40 minutes, until the fish flakes easily with a fork.

Nutritional Information

Calories: 429

Fat: 27g.

Carbs: 9g.

Protein: 37g.

Egg White Omelet

Servings: 4

Ingredients

- ✓ Cooking spray
- ✓ 2 Tbsp. onion, chopped
- ✓ 2 Tbsp. green bell pepper, chopped
- ✓ 2 Tbsp. mushrooms, chopped
- ✓ Dash of sea salt
- ✓ Dash of pepper
- ✓ 32 Oz. separated egg whites (substitutes are fine)

Directions

1. Use the cooking spray to coat a 9x5 inch glass or microwave-safe pan.

2. Sprinkle onion, green bell pepper, and mushrooms into the pan and toss it lightly with a fork. Add sea salt and pepper and then egg whites.

3. Cook in a microwave on high for approximately 3 minutes. This will vary by microwave. Remove from microwave and stir the egg whites from the side of the pan and mix with rest of ingredients.

4. Microwave for 30 to 60 seconds.

Nutritional Information

Calories: 128

Fat: 0g.

Carbs: 1g.

Protein: 25g.

Fish Soup

Servings: 4

Ingredients

- ✓ 1 Chopped onion
- ✓ ½ Chopped green bell pepper
- ✓ 2 Minced cloves of garlic
- ✓ 1 Can diced tomatoes (14 Oz.)
- ✓ 2 Cans chicken broth (14 Oz.)
- ✓ 1 Can tomato sauce (8 Oz.)
- ✓ 1 ½ Oz. fresh mushrooms
- ✓ ¼ Cup black olives, sliced
- ✓ ½ Cup orange juice
- ✓ ½ Cup dry white wine
- ✓ 2 Bay leaves
- ✓ 1 Tsp. basil, dried

- ✓ ¼ Tsp. fennel seed, crushed
- ✓ Dash of black pepper
- ✓ 1 Lb. shrimp, medium (peeled and deveined) cut into cubes

Directions

1. Start by cooking onion, green bell pepper, garlic, tomatoes, chicken broth, tomato sauce, mushrooms, olives, orange juice, wine, bay leaves, dried basil, fennel seeds, and pepper in a slow cooker for 4 hours. The vegetables should be tender, but crisp.

2. Mix in shrimp and cook for an additional 30 minutes. Remove bay leaves.

Nutritional Information

Calories: 222

Fat: 3g.

Carbs: 12g.

Protein: 31g.

Greek God Pasta

Servings: 8

Ingredients

- ✓ 16 Oz. package of whole wheat rotini pasta
- ✓ 16 Oz. can of tomatoes, peeled and diced
- ✓ 2 Tbsp. green bell pepper, chopped
- ✓ ¼ Cup green onion, chopped
- ✓ 3 Cups tomato sauce
- ✓ 1 Tsp. dried basil
- ✓ 1 Tsp. dried oregano
- ✓ 1 Cup black olives, sliced
- ✓ ½ Cup shredded mozzarella cheese
- ✓ 2 Tbsp. feta cheese, crumbled

Directions

1. Preheat oven to 400 degrees.

2. Boil a large pot of lightly salted water, and add pasta. Cook until al dente. Drain and pour into a deep casserole dish.

3. Mix tomatoes, green pepper, green onion, olives, and tomato sauce into the pasta.

4. Season with basil and oregano until it has been evenly blended.

5. Sprinkle mozzarella and feta cheese on top.

6. Bake in the oven at 400 degrees for 30 minutes.

Nutritional Information

Calories: 371

Fat: 6g.

Carbs: 68g.

Protein: 16g.

Greek Pasta and Chicken

Servings: 8

Ingredients

- ✓ 16 Oz. package linguine pasta
- ✓ ½ Cup red onion, chopped
- ✓ 1 Tbsp. olive oil
- ✓ 2 Cloves of crushed garlic
- ✓ 16 Oz. skinless, boneless chicken breast cut into bite-sized pieces
- ✓ 14 Oz. artichoke hearts, marinated and chopped
- ✓ 1 Large tomato
- ✓ 1/3 Cup feta cheese
- ✓ 3 Tbsp. fresh parsley, chopped
- ✓ 2 Tbsp. lemon juice
- ✓ 2 Tsp. oregano, dried
- ✓ 2 Wedged lemons
- ✓ Dash of sea salt

✓ Dash of pepper

Directions

1. Boil a large pot of water, and cook the pasta until it's tender. This will take approximately 10 minutes. Drain the pasta.

2. In a large skillet, heat up olive oil on medium. Add onion and garlic before sautéing. Keep sautéing until it becomes fragrant, which takes 1-2 minutes. Then stir in chicken and thoroughly cook.

3. Reduce heat down to medium-low. Add in the artichoke, tomato, feta cheese, parsley, lemon juice, oregano, and cooked pasta. Cook for an additional 3 minutes, stirring constantly.

4. Remove from heat and add sea salt and pepper. Then garnish with the lemon wedges.

Nutritional Information

Calories: 488

Fat: 11g.

Carbs: 70g.

Protein: 32g.

Greek Pasta with White Beans and Tomatoes

Servings: 4

Ingredients

- ✓ 2 Cans of Italian-style diced tomatoes (14 Oz. each)
- ✓ 1 Can cannellini beans, drained and rinsed
- ✓ 10 Oz. fresh spinach, chopped
- ✓ 8 Oz. penne pasta
- ✓ ½ Cup feta cheese, crumbled

Directions

1. Bring a large pot of water to a boil and then cook pasta.

2. While past cooks, you should cook the tomatoes and beans in a large skillet. Bring them to a boil and then reduce heat. Simmer for 10 minutes.

3. Add spinach to the sauce, and cook for 2 minutes, making sure to stir constantly.

4. Serve the sauce over pasta.

Nutritional Information

Calories: 460

Fat: 6g.

Carbs: 79g.

Protein: 23g.

Greek Potatoes

Servings: 4

Ingredients

- ✓ 1/3 Cup olive oil
- ✓ 1 ½ Cups water
- ✓ 2 Garlic cloves, chopped finely
- ✓ ¼ Cup lemon juice
- ✓ 1 Tsp. thyme, dried
- ✓ 1 Tsp. rosemary, dried
- ✓ 2 cubes of chicken bouillon
- ✓ Dash of black pepper
- ✓ 6 Potatoes, peeled and quartered

Directions

1. Preheat oven to 350 degrees.

2. Mix together olive oil, water, garlic, lemon juice, thyme, rosemary, bouillon cubes, and pepper in a small bowl.

3. Arrange cut potatoes in the bottom of a baking dish. Spread the olive oil mixture over potatoes.

4. Cover and bake for 90 to 120 minutes, turning potatoes every 30 minutes. The potatoes should be tender but firm.

Nutritional Information

Calories: 418

Fat: 18g.

Carbs: 59g.

Protein: 7g.

Grilled Banana and Peanut Butter Sandwich

Servings: 1

Ingredients

- ✓ Cooking spray
- ✓ 2 Tbsp. peanut butter
- ✓ 2 Slices whole wheat bread
- ✓ 1 Sliced banana

Directions

1. Heat a skillet on medium and spray with cooking spray.

2. Spread 1 Tbsp. of peanut butter onto each slice of bread. Then evenly place banana slices onto the peanut butter and top with the other slice, peanut butter sides facing together.

3. Cook the sandwich in the skillet until golden brown on each side. This takes approximately 2 minutes per side.

Nutritional Information

Calories: 437

Fat: 19g.

Carbs: 57g.

Protein: 17g.

Mediterranean Bean Salad

Servings: 6

Ingredients

- ✓ 15 Oz. drained can of garbanzo beans
- ✓ 15 Oz. drained can of kidney beans
- ✓ 1 Lemon, juiced and zested
- ✓ 1 Medium tomato, chopped
- ✓ ¼ Cup red onion, chopped
- ✓ ½ Cup fresh parsley, chopped
- ✓ 1 Tsp. rinsed and drained capers

✓ 1 Tbsp. extra virgin olive oil

✓ ½ Tsp. sea salt

Directions

1. Break out a large bowl, and mix together all of the ingredients. Then cover and refrigerate for approximately 2 hours, stirring every 15 minutes.

Nutritional Information

Calories: 329

Fat: 12g.

Carbs: 46g.

Protein: 12g.

Mediterranean Chicken with Eggplant

Servings: 4

Ingredients

✓ 3 Peeled and cut (lengthwise) eggplants into ½ inch. slices

✓ 3 Tbsp. olive oil

✓ 3 Diced chicken breasts, skinless and boneless

✓ 1 Diced onion

✓ 2 Tbsp. tomato paste
✓ ½ Cup water
✓ 2 Tsp. oregano, dried
✓ Dash of salt
✓ Dash of pepper

Directions

1. Soak eggplant in lightly salted water for 30 minutes to remove bitterness. Remove from water.

2. Brush eggplant lightly with olive oil. Then sauté until lightly brown.

3. Place eggplant into a baking dish and set aside.

4. Sauté the chicken and onions in a large skillet on medium. Then stir in tomato paste and water, cover and reduce heat to low. Simmer for 10 minutes.

5. Preheat oven to 400 degrees.

6. Pour the chicken and tomato mix over the eggplant. Sprinkle with oregano, salt and pepper. Cover with aluminum foil.

7. Bake in the oven for 20 minutes.

Nutritional Information

Calories: 336

Fat: 11g.

Carbs: 27g.

Protein: 35g.

Mediterranean Greek Salad

Servings: 3

Ingredients

- ✓ 3 Cucumbers, sliced and seeded
- ✓ 1 ½ Cups feta cheese, crumbled
- ✓ 1 Cup black olives, sliced and pitted
- ✓ 3 Cups roma tomatoes, diced
- ✓ 1/3 Cup sun-dried tomatoes, diced in oil (drain and reserve oil)
- ✓ ½ Red onion, sliced

Directions

1. Toss together all of the ingredients in a large salad bowl until well combined.

Nutritional Information

Calories: 131

Fat: 9g.

Carbs: 9g.

Protein: 6g.

Mediterranean Wrap

Servings: 4

Ingredients

- ✓ 1 Sliced red onion
- ✓ 1 Sliced zucchini
- ✓ 1 Sliced eggplant
- ✓ ¼ Lb. sliced fresh mushrooms
- ✓ 1 Sliced red bell pepper
- ✓ 1 Tbsp. olive oil
- ✓ Dash of sea salt
- ✓ Dash of pepper
- ✓ 4 Whole grain tortillas
- ✓ ¼ Cup goat cheese
- ✓ ¼ Cup basil pesto
- ✓ 1 Sliced large avocado

Directions

1. Place onion, zucchini, eggplant, mushrooms, and bell pepper in a container with a tight fitting lid. Sprinkle olive oil onto veggies and then season with sea salt and pepper. Close lid and shake thoroughly, mixing the veggies.

2. Heat a skillet on medium and then pour veggies onto it. Cook for approximately 10 minutes or until tender.

3. Spread 1 Tbsp. goat cheese and 1 Tbsp. pesto onto each tortilla. Divide avocados evenly on each tortilla, along with the veggie mixture.

4. Roll into snug wraps.

Nutritional Information

Calories: 436

Fat: 26g.

Carbs: 48g.

Protein: 15g.

Medley Salad

Servings: 3

Ingredients

- ✓ 4 Cups chopped raw vegetables
- ✓ 2 Oz. feta cheese

- ✓ ¼ Cup Kalamata olives, sliced
- ✓ ½ Cup basil leaves, torn
- ✓ 2 Tbsp. olive oil
- ✓ 1 Tbsp. balsamic vinegar
- ✓ Dash of sea salt
- ✓ Dash of black pepper

Directions

1. Toss all ingredients together in a large salad bowl.

Nutritional Information

Calories: 161

Fat: 12g.

Carbs: 10g.

Protein: 4g.

Melitzanes Imam

Servings: 6

Ingredients

- ✓ 1 Eggplant
- ✓ 1 Can drained diced tomatoes (14 Oz.)
- ✓ 1 Tbsp. tomato paste

- ✓ 1 Medium chopped onion
- ✓ 1 Tbsp. garlic, minced
- ✓ 1 Tsp. ground cinnamon
- ✓ 3 Tbsp. olive oil
- ✓ Dash of sea salt
- ✓ Dash of pepper

Directions

1. Preheat oven to 350 degrees.

2. Cut the eggplant in half lengthwise. Hollow out each half. Save the flesh for later use.

3. Place eggplant shells onto a baking tray, and drizzle with a small bit of olive oil.

4. Bake for approximately 30 minutes until soft.

5. While baking, cut up the eggplant flesh into small pieces. Then heat 2 Tbsp. olive oil in a skillet on medium. Cook onion and garlic for a few minutes before adding eggplant flesh. Cook until eggplant is tender.

6. Add tomatoes and tomato paste until the mixture has been thoroughly blended. Simmer on low until the eggplant shells are finished baking in the oven.

7. Remove shells and fill them with the tomato mixture. Sprinkle cinnamon on top, and then bake for an additional 30 minutes.

Nutritional Information

Calories: 314

Fat: 21g.

Carbs: 29g.

Protein: 5g.

Orzo and Chicken Salad in Red Pepper Cups

Servings: 4

Ingredients

- ✓ ½ Lb. orzo pasta, uncooked
- ✓ ¼ Cup olive oil
- ✓ 1/3 Cup red wine vinegar
- ✓ 1 Tsp. Dijon mustard
- ✓ ¾ Tsp. garlic powder
- ✓ ¾ Tsp. oregano, dried
- ✓ ¾ Tsp. onion powder
- ✓ ½ Tsp. sea salt
- ✓ ¼ Tsp. black pepper
- ✓ ½ Cup grape tomatoes

- ✓ ¼ Cup black olives, cut into halves
- ✓ 2 Oz. feta cheese, crumbled
- ✓ 1 Grilled chicken breast, cut in half
- ✓ 2 Red bell peppers, cut into halves lengthwise
- ✓ 4 Sprigs of fresh oregano

Directions

1. Add lightly salted water to a large pot, and bring it to a boil. Once boiling, stir in pasta and cook until it is tender. This takes approximately 10 minutes. Remove and drain. Let pasta cook in the refrigerator.

2. Whisk olive oil, vinegar, Dijon mustard, garlic powder, oregano, basil, onion powder, salt, and pepper in a bowl.

3. In another bowl, mix together cooked orzo, tomatoes, olives, feta cheese, and chicken breast meat.

4. Pour olive oil dressing over orzo mixture. Mix lightly.

5. Spoon mixture into red pepper halves.

6. Garnish with oregano sprig.

Nutritional Information

Calories: 462

Fat: 20g.

Carbs: 52g.

Protein: 18g.

Pan-Seared Scallops with Pepper and Onions

Servings: 4

Ingredients

- ✓ 1/3 Cup of olive oil
- ✓ 1 Can anchovy fillets, minced (2 Oz.)
- ✓ 1 Lb. large sea scallops
- ✓ 1 Large red bell pepper, chopped
- ✓ 1 Large orange bell pepper, chopped
- ✓ 1 Red onion, sliced thinly
- ✓ 1 Tsp. minced lime zest
- ✓ 1 ½ Tsp. minced lemon zest
- ✓ 1 Pinch of salt
- ✓ 1 Pinch of pepper
- ✓ 8 Sprigs parsley, fresh

Directions

1. Heat olive oil and anchovies in a skillet on medium. Stir to dissolve the anchovies.

2. Once the anchovies are sizzling, add in sea scallops, and cook for 2 minutes without moving the scallops.

3. Mix together red bell pepper, orange bell pepper, red onion, garlic, lime zest, and lemon zest in a bowl. Season this with salt and pepper.

4. Add vegetable mix to the scallops, and cook until the scallops have turned brown. This takes approximately 2 minutes.

5. Turn scallops and cook for an additional 4 minutes.

6. Garnish with sprigs and serve.

Nutritional Information

Calories: 368

Fat: 24g.

Carbs: 14g.

Protein: 24g.

Parma Wrapped Chicken with Mediterranean Vegetables

Servings: 2

Ingredients

- ✓ ½ Lb. baby red potatoes, cut into halves
- ✓ 1 Zucchini squash, cut into 1-inch slices, lengthwise
- ✓ 1 Red onion, cut into wedges, ½ inches thick
- ✓ 2 Red bell peppers
- ✓ 12 Cherry tomatoes
- ✓ 2 Tbsp. garlic, minced
- ✓ ½ Tsp. dried thyme leaves
- ✓ ¼ Tsp. red pepper, crushed
- ✓ Dash of sea salt
- ✓ Dash of pepper
- ✓ 2 Tbsp. olive oil
- ✓ 2 Skinless, boneless chicken breasts, cut into halves
- ✓ 2 Slices of thinly sliced prosciutto di Parma

Directions

1. Preheat oven to 400 degrees

2. Combine potatoes, zucchini, onion, bell peppers, and tomatoes in a bowl. Then add garlic, thyme, and red pepper to the mixture.

3. Toss until well mixed, and then add sea salt and pepper.

4. Pour olive oil onto mixture, and toss again to coat it all in the oil.

5. Pour into a glass baking dish, and bake for approximately 15 minutes.

6. Roast veggies in the oven for 15 minutes until they are tender.

7. Season chicken using sea salt and pepper. Wrap chicken breasts using the two slices of prosciutto, and secure it with toothpicks. Place it on top of the vegetable mixture.

8. Bake for about 30 minutes until the chicken is done.

9. Evenly distribute the chicken and veggies onto two plates. Cut chicken into five slices, fanning them atop of the veggies.

Nutritional Information

Calories: 570

Fat: 27g.

Carbs: 41g.

Protein: 41g.

Pasta Chickpea Salad

Servings: 6

Ingredients

- ✓ 1 Package of rotelle pasta (16 Oz.)
- ✓ 2 Tbsp. olive oil
- ✓ ½ Cup cured olives, chopped
- ✓ 2 Tbsp. minced fresh oregano
- ✓ 2 Tbsp. fresh chopped parsley
- ✓ 1 Bunch chopped green onions
- ✓ 1 Can garbanzo beans (15 Oz.) drain and rinse them
- ✓ ¼ Cup red wine vinegar
- ✓ ½ Cup Parmesan cheese, grated
- ✓ Dash of sea salt
- ✓ Dash of pepper

Directions

1. Bring a large pot of water to a boil, and cook the pasta until it's al dente. Drain and rinse pasta under cold water.

2. Heat olive oil over medium in a large skillet. Add in olives, oregano, parsley, scallions, and chickpeas. Lower heat to low, and cook for approximately 20 minutes. Place this mixture to the side and allow it to cool.

3. Toss pasta and chickpea mixture with the pasta. Add vinegar, grated cheese, salt, and pepper. Allow to chill in the refrigerator overnight.

Nutritional Information

Calories: 424

Fat: 10g.

Carbs: 69g.

Protein: 16g.

Penne with Shrimp

Servings: 8

Ingredients

- ✓ 16 Oz. Penne Pasta
- ✓ 2 Tbsp. olive oil
- ✓ ¼ Red onion, chopped
- ✓ 1 Tbsp. garlic, chopped
- ✓ ¼ Cup white wine
- ✓ 2 Cans tomatoes, diced
- ✓ 1 Lb. shrimp, deveined and peeled
- ✓ 1 Cup Parmesan cheese, grated

Directions

1. Bring a large pot of salted water to a boil, and cook pasta for approximately 8 minutes.

2. Heat olive oil in a skillet over medium heat. Add in onion and garlic, cooking until onion is tender.

3. Add wine and tomatoes to the skillet. Then cook for an additional 10 minutes, stirring occasionally.

4. Add shrimp into the skillet and cook for 5 minutes.

5. Toss mixture with pasta, and then top with Parmesan cheese.

Nutritional Information

Calories: 385

Fat: 9g.

Carbs: 48g.

Protein: 24g.

Penne with Yogurt-Tahini Sauce

Servings: 8

Ingredients

- ✓ 3 Tbsp. tahini
- ✓ 1/8 Cup lemon juice
- ✓ 1 Cup plain yogurt
- ✓ 1/3 Cup water
- ✓ 3 cloves of garlic
- ✓ ¼ Cup olive oil
- ✓ 1 Chopped onion
- ✓ 2 Sliced large Portobello mushrooms
- ✓ ½ Diced red bell pepper
- ✓ 16 Oz. package penne pasta
- ✓ ½ Cup parsley, chopped
- ✓ Dash of black pepper

Directions

1. Bring a large pot of lightly salted water to a boil, and cook pasta until al dente.

2. Mix together tahini and lemon juice. Place into a food processor along with yogurt, water, and garlic cloves. Process it until it's smooth.

3. Heat oil in a saucepan on medium. Cook onions until they are soft.

4. Add mushrooms, and continue cooking until they are soft.

5. Add bell peppers during the final few minutes of cooking so that they remain a bit crispy.

6. Drain pasta, and toss it with yogurt-tahini sauce, chopped parsley, and freshly ground black pepper.

7. Serve veggie sauce over noodles.

Nutritional Information

Calories: 332

Fat: 12g.

Carbs: 48g.

Protein: 11g.

Roasted Vegetables

Servings: 12

Ingredients

- ✓ 6 Large potatoes, diced
- ✓ 2 Diced red bell peppers
- ✓ 1 Diced fennel bulb
- ✓ 1 Diced zucchini
- ✓ 6 Cloves of garlic
- ✓ 6 Tbsp. olive oil

✓ 2 Tsp. sea salt

✓ 2 Tsp. vegetable bouillon powder

✓ ¼ Cup chopped rosemary

✓ ½ Cup balsamic vinegar

Directions

1. Preheat oven to 400 degrees.

2. Spread potatoes, peppers, fennel, zucchini, and garlic in a large baking dish. Drizzle them with olive oil.

3. Sprinkle with salt, bouillon powder, and rosemary. Stir the veggie mixture until it is well coated.

4. Bake at 400 degrees for approximately one hour, stirring occasionally. Mix vinegar into the veggies and serve immediately.

Nutritional Information

Calories: 675

Fat: 21g.

Carbs: 112g.

Protein: 13g.

Sicilian Lemon Chicken

Servings: 4

Ingredients

- ✓ ¾ Cup golden raisins
- ✓ 3 Tbsp. olive oil
- ✓ 1 Medium onion, halved and thinly sliced
- ✓ 1 Tbsp. garlic, minced
- ✓ 2 Tbsp. pine nuts
- ✓ 2 Tbsp. black olives, chopped
- ✓ 2 Bay leaves
- ✓ ¼ Tsp. oregano, dried
- ✓ ¼ Tsp. cayenne pepper
- ✓ 1 Can diced tomatoes (15 Oz.)
- ✓ Dash of seal salt
- ✓ Dash of pepper
- ✓ 1 Tbsp. balsamic vinegar
- ✓ 1 Tsp. white sugar
- ✓ 2 Tbsp. fresh basil, julienned
- ✓ 16 Oz. package of angel hair pasta
- ✓ 1 Tbsp. olive oil
- ✓ 4 boneless, skinless chicken breast halved
- ✓ 1 Lemon, juiced and zested
- ✓ ¼ Cup Parmesan cheese
- ✓ 4 Sprigs of fresh basil

<u>**Directions**</u>

1. Soak raisins in warm water until they are plump. This takes approximately 10 minutes. Drain them, and place to the side.

2. Heat 3 Tbsp. olive oil in a skillet on medium. Mix in onion, garlic, pine nuts, and olives. Season with bay leaves, oregano, and cayenne. Cook until the onions become soft. They will turn a golden brown color, which takes approximately 5 minutes.

3. Stir tomatoes, salt and pepper into mixture, and cook for an additional 5 minutes.

4. Add raisins, vinegar, and sugar. Stir and cook until it thickens, which takes approximately 5 minutes. Remove bay leaves, and add julienned basil. Cover so that it stays warm.

5. Bring lightly salted water to a boil, and cook the pasta until it's al dente. Drain.

6. In another skillet, heat up the remaining olive oil on medium. While oil heats up, mix together chicken and lemon juice. Cook chicken in skillet until it's fully done, approximately 15 minutes. Allow to cool for 5 minutes.

7. Slice each piece of chicken into thin slices, and lay it out over the pasta. Top with tomato mixture. Finally, sprinkle with lemon zest, Parmesan cheese, and a sprig of basil.

Nutritional Information

Calories: 823

Fat: 23g.

Carbs: 99g.

Protein: 57g.

Spaghetti Squash

Servings: 6

Ingredients

- ✓ 1 Spaghetti Squash, cut in half lengthwise
- ✓ Cooking spray
- ✓ 2 Tbsp. olive oil
- ✓ 3 Italian sausage links with castings removed
- ✓ 2 finely chopped spring onions
- ✓ 3 Minced cloves of garlic
- ✓ 1 Diced zucchini
- ✓ 1 Diced red bell pepper
- ✓ 1 Tbsp. Italian seasoning
- ✓ 4 Oz. crumbled feta cheese

- ✓ Dash of salt
- ✓ Pinch of lemon pepper
- ✓ 1 Finely chopped small tomato
- ✓ 1 Tbsp. fresh parsley, chopped

Directions

1. Preheat oven to 350 degrees.

2. Coat a large baking dish with cooking spray, and then place the spaghetti squash with the cut side down into the baking dish.

3. Bake at 350 degrees until the spaghetti squash is tender, which takes approximately 45 minutes.

4. Turn squash over, and bake for an additional 5 minutes. Remove from oven.

5. Scrape the squash strands into a large bowl.

6. Heat up 1 Tbsp. olive oil in a skillet over medium. Then add Italian sausage, and cook for approximately 8 minutes. Remove sausage from skillet.

7. Add 1 Tbsp. olive oil to the skillet, and cook the onions and garlic until onions are soft. This takes around 5 minutes. Then add zucchini, red peppers, and Italian seasoning. Cook for an additional 5 minutes, or until vegetables are soft.

8. Mix spaghetti squash and feta cheese with the vegetable mixture, and cook until cheese has melted.

9. Stir sausage into the mix, and season with salt and lemon pepper. Serve with tomato and parsley to serve.

Nutritional Information

Calories: 423

Fat: 30g.

Carbs: 22g.

Protein: 18g.

Spanish Cod

Servings: 6

Ingredients

- ✓ 1 Tbsp. butter
- ✓ 1 Tbsp. olive oil
- ✓ ¼ Cup onion, finely chopped
- ✓ 2 Tbsp. fresh garlic, chopped
- ✓ 1 Cup tomato sauce

✓ 15 Cherry tomatoes, cut in halves
✓ ½ Cup green olives, chopped
✓ ¼ Cup deli marinated Italian vegetable salad
✓ Dash of black pepper
✓ Dash of cayenne pepper
✓ Dash of paprika
✓ 6 Cod fillets, 4 Oz. each

Directions

1. In a large skillet, heat butter and olive oil on medium heat. Add in onions and garlic. Cook until onions are tender. Make sure you do not burn the garlic.

2. Mix in tomato sauce and cherry tomatoes. Simmer and then add green olives, marinated vegetables, and the season with a dash of black pepper, cayenne pepper, and paprika.

3. Add fillets to this sauce, and cook on medium heat for approximately 8 minutes. You should be able to easily flake it with a fork.

Nutritional Information

Calories: 170

Fat: 6g.

Carbs: 6g.

Protein: 21g.

Spinach and Feta Pita Bake

Servings: 6

Ingredients

- ✓ 1 Jar sun-dried tomato pesto (6 Oz.)
- ✓ 6 Whole wheat pita bread (6 Inches each)
- ✓ 2 Chopped Roma tomatoes
- ✓ 1 Bunch rinsed and chopped spinach
- ✓ 4 Sliced fresh mushrooms
- ✓ ½ Cup feta cheese, crumbled
- ✓ 2 Tbsp. grated Parmesan cheese
- ✓ 3 Tbsp. olive oil
- ✓ Dash of black pepper

Directions

1. Preheat oven to 350 degrees.

2. Get out the pita bread, and spread tomato pesto onto one side of each piece of bread. Place them in a baking pan, tomato side up.

3. Top bread with tomatoes, spinach, mushrooms, feta cheese, and Parmesan cheese. Drizzle on a small amount of olive oil, and then use the pepper to add seasoning.

4. Bake bread in oven for approximately 12 minutes.

5. Remove from oven, cutting the pit into quarters.

Nutritional Information

Calories: 350

Fat: 17g.

Carbs: 42g.

Protein: 12g.

Tahini Spinach

Servings: 3

Ingredients

- ✓ 10 Oz. package of chopped spinach
- ✓ ½ Cup water
- ✓ 1 Tbsp. tahini
- ✓ 2 Cloves minced garlic
- ✓ ¼ Tsp. ground cumin
- ✓ ¼ Tsp. paprika cayenne pepper

- ✓ 1/3 Cup red wine vinegar
- ✓ Dash of sea salt
- ✓ Dash of pepper

Directions

1. Add water and spinach into a sauce pan, and boil on high. Reduce to low, cover, and simmer for 5 minutes.

2. Add tahini, garlic, cumin, paprika, cayenne pepper, and red wine vinegar to a bowl and whisk. Season with sea salt and pepper.

3. Drain spinach, and then top with tahini sauce.

Nutritional Information

Calories: 69

Fat: 3g.

Carbs: 8g.

Protein: 5g.

Tilapia Feta Florentine

Servings: 4

Ingredients

- ✓ 2 Tsp. olive oil
- ✓ ¼ Cup onion, chopped
- ✓ 1 Minced clove of garlic
- ✓ 2 Bags of fresh spinach
- ✓ ¼ Cup kalamata olives
- ✓ 2 Tbsp. feta cheese, crumbled
- ✓ ½ Tsp. grated lemon rind
- ✓ ½ Tsp. sea salt
- ✓ ¼ Tsp. dried oregano
- ✓ 1/8 Tsp. white pepper
- ✓ 1 Lb. of tilapia fillets
- ✓ 2 Tbsp. melted butter
- ✓ 2 Tsp. lemon juice
- ✓ Pinch of paprika

Directions

1. Preheat oven to 400 degrees.

2. In a large skillet, heat olive oil on medium. Stir in onion and garlic. Cook for 5 minutes, until onion is golden brown.

3. Add spinach to skillet and mix down until it's wilted and cooks down. This takes 5 minutes.

4. Stir in olives, feta cheese, lemon rind, salt, oregano, and white pepper into spinach mixture. Continue cooking until cheese has melted, approximately 5 minutes.

5. Spread the spinach mixture onto a baking dish, preferably 9x13 inches. Place tilapia fillets evenly on top of the spinach.

6. Combine lemon juice and butter in a bowl, and then drizzle it over the fish. Sprinkle with paprika.

7. Bake fish at 400 degrees for 25 minutes, until it easily flakes with a fork.

Nutritional Information

Calories: 258

Fat: 13g.

Carbs: 7g.

Protein: 28g.

Tuna and Avocado Tapas

Servings: 4

Ingredients

- ✓ 1 Can white tuna packed in water (12 Oz.)

✓ 1 Tbsp. mayonnaise

✓ 3 Thinly sliced green onions (Place a small bit aside for garnish)

✓ ½ Chopped red bell pepper

✓ 1 Dash of black pepper

✓ 1 Pinch garlic salt

✓ 2 Halved and pitted avocados

Directions

1. Mix together tuna, mayonnaise, green onions, red pepper, and balsamic vinegar in a bowl.

2. Sprinkle pepper and garlic salt over mixture. Then pack the halved avocados with the tuna mix.

3. Garnish with the green onions you set aside and a dash of black pepper.

Nutritional Information

Calories: 294

Fat: 18g.

Carbs: 11g.

Protein: 24g.

Vegetable and Bread Soup

Servings: 8

Ingredients

- ✓ 1 Tbsp. olive oil
- ✓ 1 Diced large red onion
- ✓ 2 Diced carrots
- ✓ 1 Diced stalk of celery
- ✓ 4 Diced potatoes
- ✓ 10 Diced zucchini
- ✓ 1 Sliced leek
- ✓ 1 Quart of Hot Water
- ✓ 1 Chopped bunch of Swiss chard
- ✓ 1 Quartered, cored and shredded cabbage
- ✓ 1 Shredded bunch of kale
- ✓ 2 Cans of cannellini beans (15 Oz. each), rinsed and drained
- ✓ Dash of sea salt
- ✓ Dash of black pepper
- ✓ 3 Tbsp. tomato puree
- ✓ 8 Slices day-old bread

Directions

1. Heat olive oil in pan over medium. Stir in onion and cook for 5 minutes.

2. Mix in carrots, celery, potatoes, zucchini, and leek. Cook for 5 minutes, stirring occasionally.

3. Pour enough hot water into the pan to cover veggies. Mix in Swiss chard, Savoy cabbage, and kale. Reduce heat, cover, and simmer for one hour.

4. Put 1 can of the beans into a food processor and blend until smooth. Stir the pureed beans into the veggie mix, along with the second can of whole beans. Add sea salt and pepper. Reduce heat to low, and simmer for 20 minutes.

5. Add tomato paste to the mix.

6. Prepare the soup by layering the bread slices with the veggie mix in a casserole dish. Refrigerate for 8 hours.

7. Reheat soup to serve.

Nutritional Information

Calories: 352

Fat: 4g.

Carbs: 69g.

Protein: 15g.

Whole Wheat Pizza

Servings: 6

Ingredients

- ✓ 1 Whole wheat pizza crust
- ✓ 1 Jar basil presto (4 Oz.)
- ✓ ½ Cup artichoke hearts
- ✓ 2 Tbsp. kalamata olives, chopped
- ✓ 2 Tbsp. pepperoncini, sliced and drained
- ✓ ¼ Cup feta cheese, crumbled

Directions

1. Preheat oven to 450 degrees

2. Spread pesto onto pizza crust. You should use a floured surface to keep the crust from sticking.

3. Place artichoke pieces, olives, and pepperoncini evenly over pesto. Top with feta cheese.

4. Bake at 450 degrees for approximately 10 minutes, or until the crust is crisp.

Nutritional Information

Calories: 277

Fat: 19g.

Carbs: 18g.

Protein: 10g.

One Last Thing… Did You Enjoy the Book?

If so, then let me know by leaving a review on Amazon! Reviews are the lifeblood of independent authors. I would appreciate even a few words from you!

If you did not like the book, then please tell me! Email me at lizard.publishing@gmail.com and let me know what you didn't like. Perhaps I can change it. In today's world, a book doesn't have to be stagnant. It should be improved with time and feedback from readers like you. You can impact this book, and I welcome your feedback. Help me make this book better for everyone!

www.ingramcontent.com/pod-product-compliance
Lightning Source LLC
Chambersburg PA
CBHW021146260726
48656CB00024B/1607